Life's Journey

OrangeBooks Publication

1st Floor, Rajhans Arcade, Mall Road, Kohka, Bhilai, Chhattisgarh 490020
Website: **www.orangebooks.in**

First Edition, 2025

ISBN: 978-93-7426-130-9

Price: Rs. 299.00

Printed in India

LIFE'S JOURNEY

Evolve and Enhance the Experience

Dr. Tulika Jain

OrangeBooks Publication
www.orangebooks.in

Life's Journey

Evolve & Enhance the Experience

First Edition, Version 1.0

Dec,2025

Published by Dr Tulika Jain

Characters & dialogues, used to illustrate examples are from author's imagination. If there's found any resemblance to any real person or event is entirely co-incidental.

This book is dedicated-

To those who **DREAM** to become **SUCCESSFUL**

To those, who are **STRUGGLING** to get everything **PERFECT**

To those who are **SEARCHING HAPPINESS**

To those who **GOT TIRED RUNNING**, but **UNABLE TO FIND SATISFACTION** anywhere

& to the marvellous phenomenon called as LIFE

And to my parents, who always inspired me to move ahead gracefully in this journey of life …

Preface

Hi there.

Hey you, yes, I am talking to you!

How are you today?

How are you feeling nowadays?

Are you unhappy, unsatisfied, or disappointed with life?

Just take a pause before reading ahead, close your eyes, and look inside yourself.

Ask yourself this question…. How u really are?

If this question shakes you from inside, you feel a tear in your eyes either held back or dropped onto your cheeks. If you are giving a shallow smile hiding the number of compromises you are doing on a daily basis, if you are neither at ease nor at peace,

Then yes… this book is for "U."

You are not the only one who is feeling like this!!

A lot of people are perceiving the identical way – hard-luck and unsatisfied – and remain sad and uneasy every day. Continuously seek validation of others to feel happy. They are not at calm.

This book will help you to amplify your understanding about life. Delving into the depth of **Psychology**; understanding the games of mind you may experience a paradigm shift. Seeing your determination; the whole universe will guide you where you feel stuck, and will give you a hope to continue….

You may have never thought before that it's in your hand to change the experience of life!

But it's true that by throwing the dice in the right direction, **you can feel like winning rather than losing even in the same situations!**

Yes, *change in mindset through evolution - is the KEY.*

And it feels like a new birth in the same life!!

I am committed to give a helping hand to anyone who is suffering, who is in need, whoever feels restless, anxious, or unfulfilled. With an intention to enrich your life experience, I am sharing my comprehension here.

This book isn't about preaching but about walking together through life's truths. The goal isn't to fix life but to discuss some facts which are already known, but with a deeper understanding.

I believe that this book will definitely bring a positive change in your life.

"It is not the strongest of the species that survives,
It is not the most intelligent that survives.
It is the one that is the most adaptable to change."

— Charles Darwin

Introduction

Our goal in life is to be content and happy, and we spend a lot of time pursuing this happiness by chasing relationships, accomplishments, wealth, or approval. Yet something always feels missing. This is a universal truth: that despite doing "everything right", we often feel restless and incomplete. Even getting success at one step is not making us feel contented; it's just giving momentary pleasures. The next moment we again feel tangled in overthinking. Our thoughts are jumping between past regrets and future fears — creating an endless cycle of restlessness. The majority of us are worn out and irritated by this never-ending race, which makes us feel nervous and unsatisfied all the time.

We strive so much to make our life better; it still feels like life is not giving us back. Many a time we do a lot of hard work, still unable to get desired results, while sometimes we are dissatisfied with our own selves for being unable to do up to the mark.

Some people around us say, 'Be positive...' But their words irritate us in spite of transforming because they neither bring us clarity about what is positivity nor tell us how to be positive in difficult & worse situations. How can one be positive after getting continuous rejections and failures? And even if we try to be positive, the clouds of sadness don't easily leave due to the frequent bitter experiences.

So, knowing a number of challenges and various struggles, that one encounter in different stages of life, we all agree that there are enough reasons to be unhappy or sad.

Then what can you expect from this book?

In the following chapters we will discuss concepts which will assist you to unlock happiness and find contentment even in the same situations. Your perspective to see life will change; you can experience life from a broader aspect and in a much better way & yes, the sufferings will lessen!!

Here is a desire to enhance your experience of life through an evolutionary process of your mental faculty based on some psychological phenomenon & many experiences. I want you to find the source of real joy which will not only make you feel contented but also blissful.

Be determined to remodel yourself to have an experience of your favourite vehicle on the same road of life. Let's begin—

Hands-on activity: "Letter to Self"

Write a short letter to your current self – express yourself freely about what you are thinking and what you are feeling. So that at the end you can rewrite.

Contents

Chapter 1
The Restless Mind: Why We Feel Lost

It's true that there are many difficulties in almost everyone's life in today's world. There are struggling phases and uncontrollable situations that ruin one's mental peace. People are experiencing mental distress on a daily basis. They are easily agitated, gets irritable, become short tempered, later regrets, then again feel sad about everything….and this happening persistently, they get victim of depression in long run.

If this is reality, then where is the scope of improvement?

Yes, there is still a possibility, my dear, as you will go on reading, you will realize every coin has two sides. Every scene has a hidden story behind it. We are able to see till where our perception reaches. And the lights of wisdom will help you see much farther.

In this chapter, let's deepen our understanding about life process and apprehend the problem first.

Erikson's Psychosocial Theory

According to **Erikson's psychosocial theory**, there are different challenges at various stages in one's Life. **Emotional challenges begin in infancy and continue throughout life**, and unresolved conflicts at any stage often appear later as psychological distress.

In infancy, if the basic need for safety, care, and emotional warmth is not met, the individual may grow up with deep mistrust, anxiety, and fear of abandonment, which later observes as difficulty forming secure relationships.

In early childhood, when autonomy is discouraged through overcontrol or harsh criticism, the person may develop shame and self-doubt, presenting as indecisiveness, fear of making mistakes, and dependence on others' approval.

During the preschool years, if a child's curiosity and initiative are suppressed, excessive guilt may develop, which later appears as people-pleasing behaviour, suppressed anger, and fear of taking action.

In the school-age years, repeated failure, comparison, or lack of encouragement can lead to inferiority, which shows up in adolescents and adults as low self-esteem, exam fear, imposter syndrome, perfectionism, or avoidance.

Adolescence is the most critical stage for identity formation, and if this phase remains unresolved, individuals often experience persistent confusion about who they are and what they want, chronic comparison, overthinking, emotional instability, and a deep sense of being "lost," which is one of the most common issues seen today.

In young adulthood, unresolved identity and trust issues often interfere with intimacy, resulting in fear of commitment, emotional distance, relationship instability, and loneliness even within relationships.

In middle adulthood, if a person is unable to find meaning through contribution, parenting, mentoring, or purposeful work, stagnation develops, often appearing as burnout, emotional numbness, dissatisfaction despite success, or midlife crisis.

And in late adulthood, unresolved regrets and unfulfilled life meaning can lead to despair and bitterness.

Erikson's theory helps us understand that we are struggling because **a core emotional need at some stage of development remained unmet**. So, it's not totally your mistake that you are suffering. It's a chain of cause and effect.

But if this is the only truth, then there will be no option left with you other than weeping on your fate; that your needs were not appropriately fulfilled.

But according to **Adler**, unfulfilled needs occur when a person develops mistaken beliefs about themselves, others, and life. He found that **"Even if earlier needs were not fulfilled, you can choose courage, contribution, and connection now."**

I peeped into this a little more, and tried to understand why these needs developed to such an extent and remained unfulfilled also. This is because we all are thinking and behaving according to our belief system, which is developed from the existing myths about life.

Two Big Myths about Life;

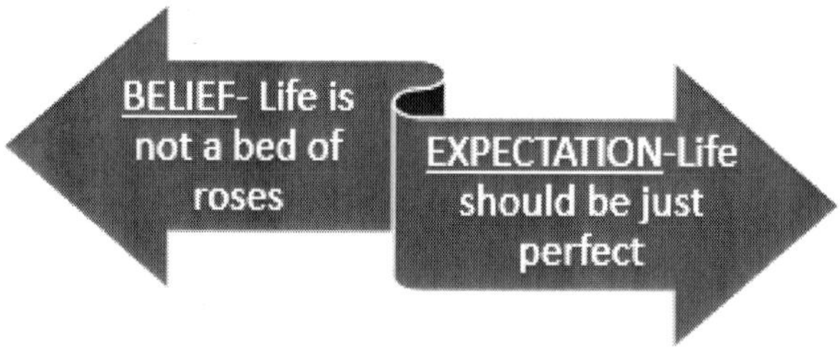

We all must have listen a famous idiom "**Life is not a bed of roses**". Some people just believe this, and no matter how much life goes in right direction, they are very sure of seeing negativity in everything. These people always focus on the dark side of things only and have already believed life is very hard.

Seema, finally became doctor and achieved her dream of wearing a white coat, but became tired of excessive hard work with constant pressure. Despite success, her journey was full of challenges. She believed that life is not a bed of roses, even after achieving big goals she was not happy.

Prabhat was nominated for a reward function; but stressed for travel expenses to reach the event in another city, having anxiety and palpitations he was continuously thinking- what if he will not be selected in final round, doubting if people will laugh at him.

Devang has got a good salaried job, but he remains sad about the tone of voice of a colleague.

People like Seema, Prabhat & Devang as in above case have accepted that life is full of difficulties, no doubt there are difficulties but they don't even focus upon points which are of so much value. It's ok to check the other side; but you are allowing only that other side to dominate your mind!

Now there exist persons with another believe "**happiness & satisfaction lies in perfect life**" They expect and strive to make life just perfect; unknowingly create pressure on themselves and when it falls a short, they feel as losing, failure, lacking, unsuccessful, unsatisfied & unhappy. Rather than enjoying life as it is, they are trapped in continuously chasing more and more. Because they expect that everything should be according to them and as it doesn't happen, they always remain sad about something.

Meera loved order.
A straight bedsheet.
A perfectly worded email.
A plan for every hour of her day.

One morning, she spilled coffee on her report-Just a few drops. But to Meera, it felt like a disaster. She threw the report and sat on the floor crying.

When Meera was a child even if she got 90%, her parent used to say- why not 95%.

She grew up believing there was only one acceptable option: **perfect or nothing.**

When you expect everything to be just perfect, even trifles are enough to disturb you. the world won't fall apart if you make a mistake but people like Meera are not living—they're surviving their own expectations.

Most of us like Meera, Seema or Prabhat in above given examples remain stressed because something is not going right in our lives? We all are Walking with a belief that life is not that easy and contradicting to our own belief we also want everything to be just perfect.

Erikson said that your emotional needs were unmet, but isn't it true **that our expectations have gone beyond reality, making our needs unquenchable?**

Let's go closer now and see why we suppose everything in life should be flawless or we get disturbed easily by small hurdles in our way.

Actually, these big myths stand upon the base of small myths that are our belief system.

Our Belief System-

These are the **silent, unconscious and rigid rules** people live by

"I must not fail." Failure=worthless. It proves I'm stupid."

"I must always be strong." Weakness = failure

"I must always please everyone." If someone is unhappy, I am bad.

"I must be perfect." "If I'm not perfect, I will be rejected."

"I must be appreciated" Criticism means I am incompetent.

"I have to constantly prove myself." If I don't succeed in areas that my parents expect- means I am not good enough.

"Everyone should take care of me" If someone leaves me, it means I am not lovable.

"Everyone should like me" they ignore me because I am not good, I'm boring."

"Everyone should agree with me" If anyone disagrees, it means I am being disrespected.

"I feel ashamed when I make mistakes". So, I avoid starting things because I'm afraid I won't do them well enough.

There is over-identification of self-worth with performance. The reason why we feel lost or restless is these set of beliefs.

These believes become **a silent operating system for life.**

"The rule that states that failure is prohibited is the issue, not the failure itself."

So, we understood till now-

Unfulfilled emotional needs at different stages of life are main cause of distress

Too much expectation of getting everything perfect is making needs unquenchable

Our hidden belief system is fabricating expectations

This loop is the root cause of generating negative emotions of anxiety and restlessness and makes us feel lost.

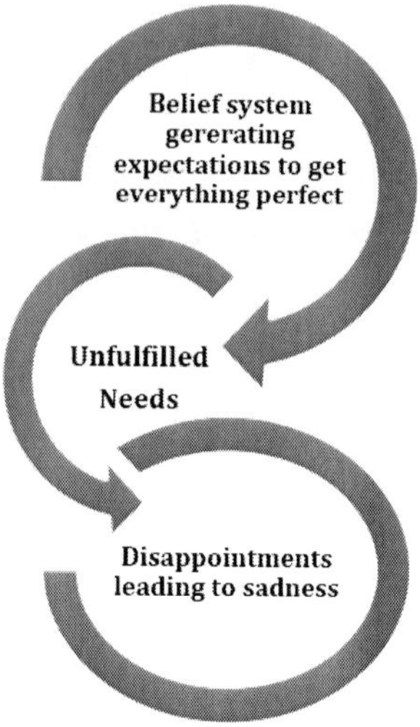

Reflection Practice

What are the top three things I keep chasing, believing they'll make me happy?

Let's dive further in next chapter to find what are factors that are making this belief system stronger and how to resolve this issue. Even after knowing the cause, is it easy to break this cycle?

Chapter 2
The Comparison Trap: How to Extricate

Snehlata, a 28-year-old girl has been married 5 years ago to a software engineer. Snehlata was very happy when her marriage was fixed to a charming person with no bad habits who used to earn a handsome salary too. He used to work at home often. These findings made Snehlata dreamt of a fulfilling luxurious & romantic life but now she looks very dull & disappointed. She is having feelings of living an unfulfilled life, as if all her dreams are broken. Because even after working from home, her husband Ramesh had no time to spend with her. She was fond of traveling while he had no desire to roam around; for him, it was a waste of money. She has to cook daily, manage home with a lot of household duties & with all these tedious works she is raising kids monotonously. She often feels to run away somewhere irritated by the children's cry and felt lonely even after everyone was present at home. This disappointment actually started since her friend's husband has posted a status on her friend's birthday, while Snehlata's husband never does that.

One of modern life's biggest causes of unhappiness—comparison.

There is an illusion created by social media, and we unconsciously measure our worth through others' success. We feel like, "Why can't my child be like her?" "Why can't my husband talk like him? "I am unable to buy car like my neighbour means my life is not good"

Movies, TV serials, and social media pics have added this unrealistic expectation in relationships. The smiley faces on social media—if you get to know them personally and about their whole life story, you will see they are not showing their silent tears on that platform; they are saying cheers only for the photographic moments, but in reality, many are suffering for one or another reason.

We have forgotten the proverb— **"The grass is greener on the other side."**

Psychologically, comparison activates feelings of inadequacy, jealousy, and anxiety because it makes us forget our individuality. It adds onto our belief—

"Others are always better than me."

"People will respect me only if I am a top performer"

"If others move ahead, I am falling behind."

Comparison doesn't exist solely- It creates a trap of complex. When you compare either you feel inferior or you feel superior, both the complexes are like a ditch. You know that if you feel inferior you immediately become sad, unsatisfied with your life situations, start doubting self-worth. But do you know that "Superiority complex" can also make you suffer!

Yes, a very common problem is not only "I am less", but also "I am above or I am the best". Actually, understand this. When you are trapped in a loop of being the best, for some time you will enjoy other people's deficiencies, but the moment they rise, you will start feeling envy, as you assume you should be the only one at the top. when you want to be better from someone else, when you strive for superiority then also you start feeling inferiority. Both the complexes walk together and in the ditch of complexes a person once fallen hinders his/her growth forever by creating constant negative thoughts.

Adler said: **“We become unhappy not because we are inadequate, but because we measure our worth by comparing ourselves with others.”**

When we compare:-

Marks

Salary

Marriage

Looks

Success

Lifestyle

We unconsciously send ourselves the message:

“I am lagging,” “I am less,” “Others are doing better than me.”

Understand this & recognize that everyone in the world is distinct and has unique qualities that do not make them better or worse. Comparison doesn't exist in nature. Sunflower has its own brightness, carnation has its own charm, rose has its own beauty & lotus has its own significance. They don't feel inferior or superior from any other of their world, they just bloom to their maximum potential.

Comparison activates the brain's reward centres, but also the pain network. When we perceive ourselves as inferior. The result: constant dissatisfaction.

Comparison also shrinks gratitude. Adler said **true mental health comes from social interest**—feeling connected, cooperative, and useful to others. And comparison does the opposite, which is another side effect of doing comparison.

It turns: -

Friends into rivals
Colleagues into threats
Relatives into competitors

Instead of connection, the person feels: Isolation, Suspicion & Emotional distance

If your happiness depends on being ahead of others, you will never be at peace, because:

Someone will always be smarter.

Someone will always be richer.

Someone will always be more successful.

Don't live a life of expectations generated because of comparison. He should say that; she should do that; my life should be like this—when these thoughts come, say to yourself that every individual is different and feels & behaves differently. To spoil your life comparing to amplified versions of social media is not worth it. You can't grow authentically while comparing your pace to someone else's. Your path is yours alone.

We have to begin to focus inward instead of competing outward. Comparison is a thief of joy—it distracts from personal growth. Instead of asking, "Why not me?", you ask, "How can I get inspired from this?" Believe in the idea of self-referenced growth: evaluating progress only against one's own past self.

Learn & evolve*: *Learn to Respect Your Individuality. Recognize that your journey has its own rhythm. Real contentment begins when one stop chasing validation and start celebrating their unique path. Inculcating self-awareness replace* *envy with inspiration and competition with compassion.*

Reflection Practice

Who do I compare myself to most?

What feeling does it create—inspiration or envy?

List three qualities you admire in others, then find three qualities that exist in you—even in small ways. This builds self-recognition and motivation.

Chapter 3
The Fear Loop: Rejection and Failure

There was a 40-year-old Bus conductor named Raju, He was of dark complexion & short height. He handled the bread and butter for his household while performing this task. Raju was not rich and used to worry about his children's future, but still things were not worse until a day when a giant-looking man sat in his bus and didn't buy the ticket. Raju was timid and didn't dare approach this man to buy a ticket because he had an angry, wrestler-like appearance. But wait, it didn't happen only for one day; this man started traveling from his bus often. Raju started having issues of trembling limbs, his sleep was gone, he used to bite his teeth in anger but didn't dare to talk to this man. Raju's mental as well as physical health started getting worse as the days were passing by; he started complaining of high blood pressure and loss of appetite. He suffered from mental restlessness.

One day Raju was down with fever and due to weakness asked his younger brother Suresh to help him in the bus. The same giant person entered the bus and unknown of the story Suresh asked him to buy the ticket. Raju started trembling with fear, thinking now his little brother would get a hit, but to his utter surprise, the giant man very politely replied that he was having a bus pass and showed some paper.

Here, Raju **experiences fear**.... which not only stops him from going ahead, but also affected his health, changing his whole life pattern. And we can assess that the fear was not real, it was fabricated inside Raju's mind due to his set of beliefs.

Yes, Life is like that.... It's not only the story of Raju but of many of us. And the problem doesn't even exist or can say exist only in our minds in forms of some anticipation.

We often underestimate our fears- take them as normal emotions and get stuck in our lives that hinders our progress.

We have to understand that **Fear is a learned pattern— built from memories and social conditioning.** These anxieties frequently stem from early life events.

<u>Our minds interpret rejection as a threat to survival and failure as proof of unworthiness.</u>

Psychologically, this happens because our brain evolved to focus on problems for survival, but now that instinct causes emotional exhaustion. The amygdala triggers fear based on past emotional memories.

See fear differently—not as an enemy but as an internal alarm trying to protect.

Realization brings calm and direction. By understanding it, you can thank fear for its intention and then gently reframe it. By naming and reframing fears, you reduce their power over behaviour and help yourself move from avoidance to courage.

We have read the famous shloka from Gita-

"Karmanye vadhika raste,
Ma phaleshu kadachana."

Here Lord Krishna also guides us to believe in ourself and instruct us to do Karma (action) without worrying about results.

When you stuck into the anticipation of results-fear of failure develops.

Fears prevent you from giving the 100%. While if you focus on the process, make strategies to handle the worse situations, learnt from past experiences-the probability to get desired result is very high.

If your mission is to get a mango tree. Sow the seed, give it proper sunlight, water, manure, follow the process, wait for the sufficient time it takes, and you will get the result the mangoes naturally.
During this process; there are chances that sudden situations like some insects, animals, cyclones may ruin it; but Its probability is very low and this is not in your control. But if you do not workout due to fear of failure, you are not going to get the fruit for sure.

If a child develops fear of falling .... What you think will happen? Will he try to move and be able to walk!? But a child is not into that loop. It develops as social conditioning is done.

Tell me if a farmer negatively anticipates about rain, and in fear of flood or drought, he doesn't harvest the crop, will you get anything to eat?

Rather than dwelling upon results working on process with a better strategy creates higher chances of getting positive outcome in life. And still if you are not getting the desired result, don't stuck into loops of fear, instead check all parameters and improve.

So, **Fear is not your enemy; it's a messenger pointing to your areas of growth. Just don't get stopped by fear instead Make a better plan guided by your fears.**

And if you are continuously not getting success in one thing, keep your eyes open may be the destiny is calling you towards something else that is meant for you. Just patiently observe, may be Universe is directing you towards something better.

Dr A P J Kalam, was rejected in the interview for Indian Air Force (IAF) pilot. Sachin Tendulkar was reported fail in his 10th-grade examinations, Pankaj

Tripathi's biggest aspiration was to own a tractor, a symbol of success in his village when he was young, but this dream remained unfulfilled, Maithili Thakur was eliminated in the early rounds of Indian Idol.

In all these cases destiny diverted them towards something bigger. Kalam Sir became one of the most popular presidents of India. Sachin Tendulkar is denoted as God of cricket. Pankaj Tripathi has become so famous for his versatile acting on the big screen. Maithili became the youngest MLA of Bihar.

Resilience is important—growth often happens when we face discomfort. Every rejection carries feedback; every failure contains wisdom.

Through real-life reflections, courage isn't the absence of fear but the willingness to move forward despite it. Believe in yourself. Sincerity and diligence are never in vain. Destiny is waiting for you- Just keep going.

Stop lingering on fear of failure. You must be empowered to act, not held back by imagined limitations. You won't fall into the vicious cycle of rejection and failure if you don't care about the outcome. Many times, the problem is just imaginary thus it's important to work upon the process in order to accomplish any goal. Trust that by following proper strategy, outcome is inevitable.

So, in this chapter we analysed three major questions-

- Why we have fears?
- How fears can hinder our growth?
- How to use fears as a friend rather than enemy

Learn & evolve*: *Reframe failure as feedback and rejection as redirection in your belief system. Shift from "What if I fail?" to "What if I learn?" Plan and follow a discipline, if fail-learn and try again. Fear loses power when you face it with curiosity instead of avoidance.*

Reflection Practice

What do I fear most right now?

What's the story my mind talks about this fear?

Hands-on activity

Use the "What if it goes right?" technique. Each time a fear appears, ask yourself what positive outcome could also be possible. Write both side by side.

Chapter 4

The Illusion of Control: Confrontation with Reality

Priyanka is just 30 years old, but she is feeling completely lost after being unable to clear the Civil Services exam. She has given many years in preparation but without any positive outcome. Now she feels she is not good enough. She doesn't know what she will do in life now. Since the results were announced, she has shut her room and stopped communicating with anyone. She is very angry at her aunt, who just commented on her results when she was entering the room & feeling worthless at the same time.

Most people who lead a disappointed life, feel that they are unable to live a life they want.

They are unable to get selected in their desired stream.

Their relationships are not able to meet their expectations.

Their boss is not appreciating them.

Their juniors are not listening, not giving respect to them.

Their business is not giving the desired outcome.

Their family is not supporting them.

They are not able to control their emotions.

They are unable to make the money they wanted.

& they mark themselves as a failure

You can say they are absolutely right; when things are not going the way they wanted, it's obvious that they feel depressed.

Heyyyyyyy wait wait wait.

Here is a big delusion. Who said you—that your life will go exactly the way you wanted?

Ok, let’s review, there are only 10 seats in an entrance exam; and 100 candidates. So is it possible that life go according to all 100 people. Obviously NO- even if they all are intelligent, all are hardworking, all are deserving then also, 90 people have to face disappointment because seats are just limited. You know all this and still when the results are announced, you start suffering!!

We think that we can control everything, and when we can't, it leaves us in a gloomy state.

You have to understand what can and what cannot be controlled.

In the above case Priyanka should realise that only doing efforts is in her hands, not the results. And she cannot control what her aunt or anyone says. Maybe if today, she cleared this exam, she may fail at another promotion of life. Understand that today aunt has said something bitter but even if she talked sweetly, may be tomorrow any other higher officer behaves rudely with her, if she got admission; there are chances that seniors might say something, if not there, after getting job boss may say something. And you can't control everything. The only Solution is having a deep understanding of life's journey. If you are predicting and expecting things to happen only your way then definitely you are living with a false belief. Either today or tomorrow, its high possibility that you will get disappointed.

Psychologically, control is rooted in fear — fear that if we don't manage everything, things will fall apart. The truth, however, is that peace comes when we let go of what's beyond us and focus on what's within us: our thoughts, choices, and responses.

So, when you know this fact, how does not getting a seat define you? Please stop living in a dream world. You are a human being with a large logical brain, use its functioning in analysing and making a better world for you. Don't let its part of emotion damage your life. Emotions will come, but use them to direct your life in a better way. When we try to control everything — outcomes, people, emotions—end up exhausted. This makes us irritable, and further turn into anger with rage. They take away your mental peace and leave you distracted from your path. Sometimes these emotions develop into hatred which later affects the physical health resulting into diseases like diabetes, hypertension etc.

Even Many people regret after their reaction but can't help. These people give reason for their behaviour that this person in front did such thing, or that person talked in a disgraceful manner or didn't work properly as they wanted. But actuality is, by showing anger you try to control everything in your hand. You want that people around you should behave according to you and should perform exactly as you want.

We overestimate control to reduce uncertainty. When matters don't go our way, we suffer. We cling to control circumstances — because uncertainty scares us. But life, by nature, is uncertain. trying to control everything only breeds anxiety, while acceptance brings peace. And acceptance is not resignation, but a freedom —it's the art of letting go gracefully. Guys, you have to come out of this illusion that everything can be controlled, then only you will be able to break this process which lead you towards an unhappy, unsatisfied life-

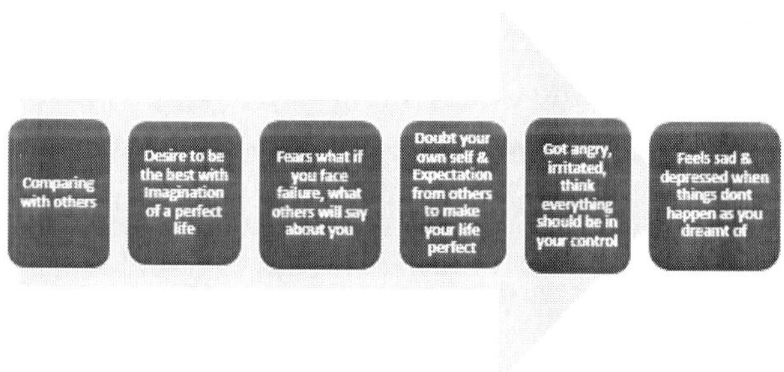

Neha and Priya both lost their jobs when their company suddenly shut down. The event was exactly the same. The shock was the same. The uncertainty was the same. But what happened inside their minds was completely different.

That night, Neha kept thinking,

“I have failed in life. I’ll never be successful. Everyone will look down on me. I don’t know what I’m doing with my life.”

These thoughts ran in a loop. As a result, she started feeling **hopeless, anxious, and lost**. Within a few days, she stopped applying for jobs, stayed in bed most of the time, avoided people, and kept saying, “What’s the point?”

Neha was not suffering mainly because of the job loss—she was suffering because of her **automatic negative thoughts**: When situations were not under her control she started feeling- *I am a failure, my future is ruined, and nothing will work out.*

Priya also felt scared that night. But her thoughts were different. She told herself,
"This is just a hurdle, yet not the end of my existence." I’ve handled difficulties before. I’ll take some time, update my skills, and apply again.”
Because her thoughts were more balanced, her emotions were different too. She accepted life as is; she felt **worried but hopeful**, sad but motivated. Within a week, she updated her resume, contacted old colleagues, and started planning her next steps.

Both faced the **same external situation**—job loss.

Neha felt lost because **her thoughts told her that the situation was permanent, personal, and hopeless.**

Priya stayed emotionally stable because **her thoughts framed the situation as temporary, manageable, and meaningful for growth.**

Adler said we are driven by an unconscious life goal.

Neha's hidden goal seems to be:

→ *"I must never fail to have value."*

When failure happened, her entire meaning system collapsed.

Priya's life goal appears to be:

→ *"To grow, adapt, and become stronger."*

So even failure became part of her progress.

When two people face the same difficult situation—such as failure, uncertainty, breakup, or career setback—and yet one feels completely lost while the other remains emotionally steady, **Adler** explains this difference through the purpose they choose further. He said people act based on **private logic**, not objective reality, developed according to their own **Hidden Belief System.**

The Belief System Filter

Our life is progressing according to our set goals, which are formed according to the belief system that life should be perfect, everything should go my way, it's very hard to get success, and I should never fail to get appreciation & recognition.

Every person views situations through internal "filters":

People who believe mistakes equal failure → panic

People who believe mistakes equal learning → growth

These filters were shaped by past experiences, feedback, and personality.

Now it's in our hand to bring changes in our life by changing our belief system.

Thus, if we change our belief system and accept & start enjoying whatever is there, in spite of the same circumstances, the suffering can be reduced. By understanding the reason behind the suffering, we can evolve our lives to a great extent. So, even if you had a bad past experience, you know that circumstances are not under your control but your happiness is!

Learning acceptance rewires emotional regulation and increases adaptability.

Release this illusion of control with a belief that surrender is not weakness but wisdom.

Through acceptance, we conserve energy and open ourselves to creative solutions.

Learn to trust life more — not blindly, but consciously.

You can't control life's flow, but you can control how you surf its waves.

Learn & evolve**—** *Don't live in the illusion that you can control everything; rather, you can direct your life in every circumstance you go through. From this moment onwards you can decide to live a happier life.* ***Peace begins where control ends.

Reflection Practice

What recent event frustrated me because it didn't go my way?

Hands-on activity

Draw two circles: one labelled "What I Can Control," the other "What I Can't." Fill them honestly. Focus only on actions inside your control circle for one week.

So now when we know the reason for getting frequent disappointments, in the next chapter Let's peep further what are other hurdles in the way of happiness and what's stopping us from moving ahead…

Chapter 5
Confined in Overthinking: Here's the Solution

Shweta is a 24-year-old postgraduate student. She was brilliant in studies in junior classes but soon she felt into trap of overthinking, her focus on studies were gone. If her teacher looks serious in class, she keeps thinking, *"Did I say something wrong?";* When a friend responds slowly, she considers "Maybe I offended him,". She spends hours replaying even the smallest errors she makes in assignments, in her mind.

Before sleeping, her thoughts jump into the future: *"What if I fail? What if I don't get a job? What if people think I'm useless?"* She complained that every time she sits to read something, the flood of thoughts starts coming into her brain, which she just can't help and later when no time is left, she used to regret a lot. She often blames herself also for this overthinking; which only increased her thoughts further.

Amit is a 32-year-old software professional working in a private firm. He is sincere, punctual, and technically capable. But mentally, he is always tense. Before clicking "send," he reads each email at least three or four times. "Was my tone correct?" he still wonders, even after sending it. *Did I sound rude or incompetent?"* During meetings, if his manager casually says, "We'll discuss this later," Amit's mind starts racing: *"Did I say something wrong? Are they unhappy with my performance? Will this affect my appraisal?"* If a colleague gives neutral feedback, he interprets it negatively.

If someone does not greet him warmly, he spends the entire day analysing possible reasons. At home, instead of relaxing, his mind replays office conversations like a recorded tape. Soon Amit reached a breaking point when he started having frequent headaches, disturbed sleep, and constant chest tightness before office meetings.

Thinking

Thinking

Overthinking

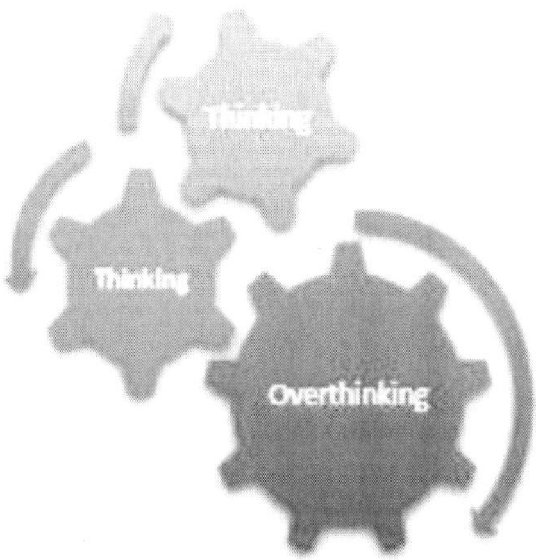

Many people say, that they overthink, and they again think about it that they are overthinking and feels bad about it. They find it difficult to come out of this bush, which is very dense, and they feel tangled.

Who can overthink?

Firstly, understand one thing: **who can overthink?** Is it possible for any non-living thing to think or even all living creatures can an ant, or a butterfly or a flower get involved into this process?

No, it's you, the human being, who possesses this extraordinary strength and quality. The human being could invent so wonderful & amazing things only because of this capability of thinking. The more you are capable of thinking means, your brain is working so efficiently. We all are actually blessed to have this power.

But what happening is, people are feeling crazy because of the overcrowding of thoughts and because they are unable to stop them.

Why we Overthink?

Cognitive Behavioural View explains overthinking as a result of **distorted thinking patterns**, such as:

Catastrophizing: “Something terrible will happen.”

Mind reading: “They must be judging me.”

Overgeneralization: “This always happens to me.”

These distorted thoughts keep triggering emotional stress, which fuels more thinking.

Another reason is suppression of emotions like anger, sadness, guilt, or grief. When these are not expressed, the brain converts emotional pain into mental noise. Overthinking becomes the mind’s way of processing what the heart could not express.

And it eventually becomes addicting due to the brain's dopamine loop. The brain mistakenly believes, "Thinking more will give relief." But instead of relief, it creates more stress, which again triggers more thinking—a classic mental addiction loop.

In One Line: Overthinking is the mind's attempt to protect you from future pain using thought—but when fear controls the mind, protection becomes torture.

Shweta & Amit are not weak-minded. They are fear-driven, self-doubting, and perfectionistic—the exact emotional soil where overthinking grows.

What's the solution?

So, what you have to do now; what's the solution to come out of this bush?

Overthinking does not disappear by force.

You can't stop thinking, but you can give them a healthy direction.

Understand this by some Examples-

1. Your boss says, "We'll talk later."

Overthinking:

"I'm in trouble. What is he going to say now! Will he scold me? I must have messed up. I'll lose my job."

Healthy thinking:

"It could be about many things. I'll wait and handle it when it comes."

2. You made a small mistake at the workplace.

Overthinking:

"I'm so careless. Everyone will think I'm incompetent. This will ruin my image."

Healthy thinking:

"Mistakes happen. I'll correct it and move on."

3. Someone looks serious while talking to you.

Overthinking:

"They're angry with me. I must have said something wrong."

Healthy thinking:

"They may be dealing with their own stress. It's not necessarily about me."

4. Friend doesn't reply to your message.

Overthinking:

"They're ignoring me. I must have upset them. Nobody really values me."

Healthy thinking:

"They might be busy. I'll wait or follow up later."

Overthinking reduces when:

Control is replaced by acceptance

And self-criticism is replaced by self-compassion.

You won't ever suffer from your ideas if you have a deep comprehension of the situation.

Learn & evolve- Overthinking is not an issue at all when you have a healthy thought process; which is developed when Fear is replaced by self-trust!*

Hands-on activity

Gently ask yourself: "What is my mind worrying about right now?"

Separate Thought from Reality by slowly repeating in your mind:

"This is a thought… not a fact."

Practice this daily.

So, now when you have got a solution for your overthinking and you are not going to get effected by it any more in next chapter let's see how changing the lens through which we view life; can completely alter our experience.

Chapter 6
The Power of Perspective: Rewrite the Inner Story

While looking out of the train's window, I was seeing roads, farms, trees, mountains, and stations all passing by one by one. Some views were just of simple houses alongside the track; some were exceptionally beautiful scenes of nature. At one moment there were pleasant sights of lakes; at another, also dirty drains. It was a long trip, and I was thinking **life is also a journey where different stages just pass by one by one, giving variable experiences.**

Even it's also possible that some tracks follow only unpleasant sites or some take you along only the wonderful ones. As the life's journey is different for all individuals. But as I noticed – a fighting couple in one coach, a romantic couple in another coach, a crying child at one birth, a dancing kid at another, an old couple enjoying their home food in one section, an old person distressed with his knee pain in another, a group of friends playing cards together at one place, some people disputing politics at another – a second thought clicked in my mind: even if two people are facing the same situation, is it possible that both may experience it from a different viewpoint?

Ayaan and Rakesh worked in the same office.

One morning, their manager called them in and said,

"Your presentation last week had several mistakes. Both of you need to revisit it and make further improvements."

They left the room together—but what happened inside their minds changed everything.

Same words.
Same tone.
Same moment.

But the rest of their day?
Completely different.

Ayaan's Inner Dialogue- As they walked out, Ayaan's thoughts started racing:

"I messed up again."
"Everyone must think I'm incompetent."
"Why can't I ever get things right?"

Because of these thoughts, Ayaan avoided everyone the whole day.

He didn't ask his manager for clarification.

He worked alone, stressed and panicked… and made even more mistakes.

By evening, he felt exhausted and defeated—not because of the manager's words, but because of the *story he told himself.* Rather than feeling worse, he could have ended up learning something.

Rakesh's Inner Dialogue- Rakesh heard the exact same feedback, but his inner voice was different:

"Okay, mistakes happen."
"It's not a judgment on my value; it's just feedback."
"What exactly needs fixing? I can learn this."

He took a deep breath. He felt alert, not anxious.

He asked his manager for specifics.
He discussed ideas with teammates.
He corrected the document methodically, even adding new insights.

By evening, he felt motivated and proud—not because the situation was easy, but because of the *story he chose to believe*. His inner dialogue became his strength.

So, yes, it is possible that different people on the same track may experience the journey differently!!

In the above given example we saw,

Two people.

One situation.

One powerful difference.

What caused these two completely different responses?

Cognitive Appraisal Theory says- it's not the event that causes emotion—it's how we interpret the event.

Ayaan interpreted the manager's words as a *threat to his self-worth.* Inner dialogue was self-blaming, which led to stress, avoidance, and poor performance.

→ Emotion: anxiety, shame

→ Behaviour: withdrawal, avoidance

Rakesh interpreted the same words as *information to improve.* Inner dialogue was curious and balanced, which led to clarity, confidence, and action.

→ Emotion: motivation

→ Behaviour: problem-solving, engagement

Self-talk directly influences the amygdala (fear centre in your brain) and the prefrontal cortex (thinking centre in your brain):

Negative self-talk activates the amygdala, causing stress and fight-or-flight behaviour.

Balanced or positive self-talk activates the prefrontal cortex, enabling clarity and problem-solving.

So, Ayaan's thoughts triggered fear.
Rakesh's thoughts triggered focus.

Every person lives inside a story they tell themselves—

"I'm not good enough." "I can't change," "This is my fate," which further makes us believe that I am done now, I am tired now, I don't have time, I can't make much money, I am useless, people are not happy with me, & so on.

Just imagine the change in our lives if we change these inner dialogues with "I am enough", "Every individual is unique", "I have my own pace and timeline". "I can create my own destiny"

And it is not difficult to write this inner story.

Do you remember the quotations we have read & heard since our childhood.
"Be kind to oneself & others" "Hope is life." "Time is money," "Change is the only constant," etc.

Friends, those little quotations even hold enormous power, like an atomic bomb. Because they will alter your belief system if you comprehend and comply. However, we see them as merely a proverb to jot down in our diaries, and we create our own inner quotations that state that there are problems in life at every turn.

And why does it happen? – Because the Brain Is Built for Survival, Not Happiness

Problems feel urgent → the brain zooms in.

Solutions feel optional → the brain postpones them.

Your mind isn't being "negative"—it's being *protective.*

Identify the inner narrative that drives self-doubt, as these unconscious narratives are shaping your emotions and behaviours. & use self-compassion, affirmations, and psychological reframing to rewrite these tales.

Believe in the concept of cognitive reframing—the process of replacing limiting beliefs with empowering truths.

Nothing in the outer world changed.

Their inner world shaped their feelings, and their feelings shaped their behaviour.

Your inner dialogue is not just a talk- It is the glass filter through which you observe the world. Change the lens, and the experience changes with it.

*Learn & Evolve**

✨ *You may not control the situation, but you can always control the conversation inside your mind.*

✨ *And when you change that inner dialogue, you change your emotions.*

✨ *When you change your emotions, you change your actions.*

✨ *And when you change your actions… you change your life.*

Key Takeaway

You are not your thoughts—you are the author who can rewrite them. The goal is to question your thoughts, not obey them.

"Cultivate a positive mental environment, as you dedicate the majority of your existence there."

Till now you understood, that You live according to your inner dialogue — change the story, and your reality transforms. Perspective is everything. As of now, you are on the path of self-awakening, understanding the games of your mind. Let's discuss in the next chapter how to play the dice of success!

Chapter 7
Redefine Success: 'Vincit qui Patitur'

Rohit and Aman both failed the same competitive exam. They had studied in the same coaching class, faced the same paper, and received the same result— **"Not Selected."**

That evening, Rohit sat alone in his room, staring at the wall. His mind kept repeating,
"Everyone is moving ahead. I am stuck. What is the point of my life now?"
Within days, he stopped talking to friends, avoided books, and began feeling lost and empty. For Rohit, this failure didn't just mean an exam loss—it felt like a **loss of identity**. Deep inside, he had always believed, *"If I don't succeed, I am nothing."* So,

when success didn't come, his sense of self collapsed.

Aman also felt sad that evening. He talked to his parents, went for a walk, and said,
"Yes, this hurts… but this is not the end."
A week later, he started planning again—another attempt, another path, maybe even a new field. Aman's belief was different: *"Failure is painful, but it doesn't decide my worth."* He still felt disappointed, but he did not feel lost.

Both faced the **same failure**.
Rohit felt lost because his **entire identity was tied to success**.
Aman stayed emotionally stable because his **identity was stronger than the situation**.

According to **Alfred Adler**, success has a very different meaning from the common idea of achievement, status, or winning.

For Adler, **success is not about being above others—it is about contributing to others.**

He believed humans are healthiest and happiest when they use their abilities to benefit others, create connection, and improve the community.

Society teaches us to equate success with luxury, fame, and constant achievement, yet those often bring temporary satisfaction.

Try to see what success truly means. Define success internally—through peace, authenticity, and meaningful relationships.

Liberate yourself from peer-driven expectations and social pressure, and rediscover true ambition.

Define success in your own terms—not by wealth or luxury, but by inner peace and alignment.
"Vincit qui patitur" is a Latin phrase meaning **"he who endures conquers."**

When you feel being successful means this particular seat or post or position—just ask yourself, "Will all your life struggles end once you get that seat?

No—only their form will change."

Setting objectives is beneficial and crucial, but it's important to have mental clarity that what you actually want???

And there will be UNLIMITED OPTIONS, because your goal is not based on narrow thinking but a broad perspective, which is in alliance with this universe & You will explore how intrinsic goals (personal growth, learning, connection) bring lasting fulfilment, while extrinsic ones (status, money, image, position) are never enough.

Realise you don't need to run faster—you need to walk in the right direction. Release the pressure to "catch up" and instead focus on living purposefully and peacefully.

We also often feel successful when we get something, like respect from others, love from our relationships, gifts on our special days, appreciation by authorities. We define in our mind that if we get these things, it means we are successful; getting these norms fulfilled will make me happy …. And when we don't get these… we feel unsuccessful, leading to feelings of sadness & depression.

But

If

U

Ask me.

The SECRET… ONLY ONE LINE… IF YOU CAN UNDERSTAND THIS

What You Give—You Get

We always want from others…. Happiness, gifts… and even friendship… love

Don't keep waiting for others to give you…

Just make a change in your moves—start thinking about what you can give and not what you can get—and see the miracle of how successful you will be, not only in one but in every aspect of life.

Start thinking about what you can give and not what you can get.

Psychological Insight

Extrinsic goals (money, fame, rewards) activate dopamine but fade quickly; intrinsic goals (growth, connection) create long-term satisfaction through serotonin and oxytocin release.

Two students, A and B, study for an exam.

Student A (ego-driven):

“I have to top the class. If someone does better, I’m a failure.”

Student B (Adlerian mindset):

"I want to learn well in order to become a good doctor and to help society."
Both study hard.

But only B finds meaning, satisfaction, and long-term growth.

According to Adler, **B is successful**—not because of marks, but because of *purpose and contribution.*

And as stated in last chapter, another point of view is- in spite of pondering upon results, start giving your time & focus to books—you will also get good marks, will get selected and will be able to become a good doctor and help society as well!

A Story of a Boy Who Fixed the Light

In a small town, there was an old library that everyone loved.
Children came there after school, elders came for newspapers, and students came to study late into the evening.
One winter, the main reading room light stopped working.
It flickered all day, then finally went dark.
People complained:

"How can we read now?"

"The librarian should fix it."
"The government never maintains anything."
Everyone waited for someone else to solve the problem.

Among these voices was a 17-year-old boy named Arjun.
He wasn't the topper in school, he wasn't the best athlete, and he often felt invisible among his classmates.

But that evening, he quietly walked to the librarian and said,
"Can I try to fix the light? My father is an electrician. I've helped him many times."
The librarian smiled gently.
"Of course, beta. Go ahead."
Arjun climbed on a stool, checked the wiring, cleaned the holder, and replaced the old tube, and within minutes—

The reading room lit up bright.

People looked up smiling.
An old man said, "Arjun, thank you. Now I can read my newspaper properly."
A small girl clapped and said, "Yay! I can finish my storybook!"
The librarian put a hand on his shoulder and said,
"You helped everyone today."

Arjun felt a warmth he had never felt before.

Not pride… but **belonging**.

Not superiority… but **usefulness**.

Walking home, he realised something important:

He hadn't become smarter than others.
He hadn't competed with anyone.
He hadn't proved he was "the best".
But he had **contributed**.
He had used his small skill to make life better for everyone around him.

And he felt **successful**.

Not because he outshone someone,

But because he **made a difference.**

Learn & evolve*

- *Success is peace of mind—alignment between who you are and what you do.*
- *Success is measured in contribution, not competition.*
- *Success is self-improvement for cooperation, not self-improvement for domination.*
- *The one who has the courage to take imperfect steps is already successful.*
- *Success is when your goals serve life, not just your ego.*

Reflection Practice

What version of success was I taught to chase?

What truly makes me feel fulfilled?

Write your personal success statement:

Key Takeaway

You're not behind; you're just not meant to follow someone else's path.

Success is not standing above people; it is standing with people and being useful to them.

"Having the firmness to elevate oneself and have a favourable influence on the world is the key to triumph."

Now that you have redefined success for yourself, see how beautifully contentment follows your way in the next chapter…

Chapter 8
Contentment: Your New Companion

Jai is a 37-year-old guy with an office job from 10 to 6. His boss is very rude to him. Jai feels that there are very bad politics running in the office, as he has not been promoted to the next level even after working so hard. He wants to leave the job but is not getting any better opportunity in the same city. He doesn't want to change the city because of Parent's responsibility. His wife also shouts many times for his careless attitude. He constantly remains restless; life has just become a burden for Jai, and he doesn't remember when the last time was that he felt happy and satisfied!

Prakash is now 50 years old. He purchased a house sometime back and now remains in constant worry about paying the EMIs. He is doing overtime, searching for multiple work opportunities to earn more money, but health is not giving him a green flag. His doctor is advising him not to work more. So, he is unable to sleep and suffering from restless nights with insomnia.

You may feel after reading this that yes, there are enough reasons to be discontented with Jai & Prakash.

And with your life also, you can recall so many things to be dissatisfied about.

But pause & reflect; let's see this from a different angle…

In Jai's case, definitely there are situations which can trouble anyone, but let's analyse without being biased, without fixing life at its harder side. At least Jai has a job, which puts him in a much better situation than many unemployed persons. His job is only 10-6, which allows him to devote meaningful time to his family as well as personal care and interests. His body and brain are working so well; that is why he is expecting a promotion. He is taking on a parent's responsibility; that means he is a dutiful person and must be getting affection & blessings from elders. He has a wife who cares for him, and that's why she points out his mistake so that he can be a better person. He doesn't know exactly what is happening in management; it's only assumed that there are some unfair favours. Even if there is politics, if Jai starts focusing on his work, he may get a promotion as well in the coming time, as every individual possesses unique capabilities which are irreplaceable, and even if he doesn't get one, there are enough things with him to have a wonderful experience of life.

In the second case of Prakash also, after seeing another side of the coin, we can tell him, 'You are paying EMIs; that means you own a house, which is still a dream of many.' You are doing work; that means you are capable. You are consulting a doctor; that means you can still afford the fees. The doctor is suggesting a therapy that means whatever illness you have can be improved.

But the reasons- why people like Jai & Prakash are unable to see from this angle! - we had already discussed in previous chapters.

Because they already assume that life is not a bed of roses, and at the same time, they want everything to be perfect. They think everything should be in their control, but forget at the same time –boss, parents, wife or husband, colleagues, and everyone else- also want them to be their way!

And by running after perfection, they start looking at those points which are imperfect. It's like seeing only the black spots on a white paper. Now the focus on deficiencies makes them feel lacking; this feeling reduces mood. With a low mood, the behaviour and action are affected, and this triggers the life events to be even worse. And the cycle goes on.

If you realise all of our minds are constantly racing comparing — regretting, predicting — and that constant mental noise disconnects us from peace. There's a pattern of overthinking and emotional chaos in almost every case. Reflect on how life becomes lighter when we stop fighting it and start understanding it. worrying about a mistake, replaying conversations, or comparing progress — but awareness breaks the loop.

Now it's your choice: focus on the dark side and keep lamenting, or focus on both sides equally, enjoy the goods in your life, and make a plan to manage the rest.

Remember that we all are mortals; we have a vulnerable aspect of life. As we age, by a very

natural process, physical health declines. We can't control everything, but we can take care as much as we can.

In every corner of the world right now, people are wandering discontented and unsatisfied with their lives-

On one side the poor are struggling for their physiological needs; on the other side the rich are struggling for psychological needs.

A failed student is harassed by his parents or teachers, while a top student is facing a lot of self-mental pressure to keep up his image & position in society.

A lady who is working herself at home feels overworked and tired, whereas a lady who has a helper maid is stressed because she is not getting the perfect work done.

An unemployed man feels he is good for nothing, while the person at the job is feeling used by his management.

Someone is unable to find a right partner and remains unmarried; someone is not satisfied with his/her partner.

The mind always wants "more." creating dissatisfaction even in abundance.

Contentment means a deep sense of inner satisfaction and peaceful acceptance of what you have, who you are, and where you are in life.

Contentment doesn't say you stop trying to improve; it just says don't suffer while you struggle, accepting it as a process of growth.

Contentment strengthens with awareness. Joy is not in reaching the destination but in being awake to the journey itself. Gratitude, mindfulness, and presence can quiet the inner chaos.

Note: Here you must acknowledge one thing: I do not suggest focusing only on the bright side either, because it will work only for some time; after that, you will start feeling that you have deluded yourself. Always remember a coin has two sides, and you have to consider both.

Contentment is not complacency — it's the art of appreciating what is; while still growing.

Contentment grows where appreciation lives.

It is a calm state where: -

- ✓ You appreciate the present.
- ✓ You feel "enough" inside.
- ✓ You are not ruled by comparison.
- ✓ You are not chasing happiness outside yourself.

Now the question is-

IF I AM AMBITIOUS- MEANS AM I GREEDY?

DO CONTENTMENT MEANS- I SHOULD NOT ASPIRE FOR GROWTH AND REMAIN SATISFIED WHERE I AM?

& the answer is NO- it is not so

BEING CONTENTED DOESN'T MEAN THAT YOU LOWER YOUR GOALS OR GIVE UP ON GROWTH

Rather it emphasises you to transform on following points while travelling the path of growth-

- ★ **At times of failure- Speak kindly with yourself**

- ★ **Make peace with whatever you cannot control**
- ★ **Accept imperfection courageously**
- ★ **Shift from comparison to belonging**
- ★ **Understand contentment lives now not later**

The true satisfaction follows you everywhere in your path when there is the inner harmony that comes when a person feels useful, connected, and socially contributing

And Simple awareness of small joys — a breath, a meal, a conversation —awakes deep happiness.

A One-Line Formula for Contentment

Contentment = Acceptance of the present + Contribution to others + Compassion toward self

Psychological Insight

Gratitude practices increase serotonin and rewire the brain's attention system to focus on abundance instead of lack.

Learn & evolve* *Shift your focus from deficiencies to blessings that you have. Accept the imperfections. Learn that contentment is now and not in future.*

Now with a contented soul, let's add some more joy as we walk towards conclusion….

Chapter 9
Encounter Evolution: Experience the Joy of Living

I *know that you are already repeating the below lines in your mind-*

I have evolved* From now onwards I will never ever compare myself with anyone. Rather, I will enjoy the process of improving myself. ☺

I have evolved* From now onwards I will set goals but not ponder about results. If some anticipatory anxiety occurs, and some fears come up, I will observe them and use them to make my plan better but never allow any fears to stop me. Even after that, if failure occurs, rather than sitting hurt, I will try to learn & try again with more precise steps. I will be open-minded and will try to see the various opportunities even in adverse situations. ☺

I have evolved * From now onwards I will never react to someone's activity which I don't like, because it's not necessary that everyone speak or act according to me. I will also not get affected by any negative outcome for which I worked hard; surely, I can feel sad for some time as I am a sensitive human being, but I will not let these emotions stay for long or turn into a gloomy state because now I know the fact of limitations in every field. Now I know I can only try, but I can't control everything. ☺

I have evolved* From now onwards I will never be affected by overthinking. Now I know it's my power to think and by directing it towards healthy thinking, I will use it to make my life better. ☺

I have evolved* From now onwards I will choose the words very wisely, that I say to myself-because now I know my inner story can change my outwardly experience. ☺

I have evolved* From now onwards I have amplified my belief system- redefined success for me. I will not chase perfection but work upon kaizen i.e. continuous improvement ☺

I have evolved* From now onwards contentment is my new companion as I now understand what really contentment means. It doesn't hinder my growth but makes my journey of growth pleasurable! 😇 ☺

These key points are like blessings to live a happy & contented life!!

Live your life guided by these convictions- and your sufferings will significantly reduce. You will be able to live a successful and contented life.

Now, let me share with you, another pearl of wisdom by delving into an extensive insight about life which will not only help you to find the ultimate source of joy but also make you peaceful with your journey!

Abraham Maslow has given a theory explaining **what humans need to feel fulfilled**, arranged in a pyramid from the most basic to the highest psychological growth known as **"Maslow's Hierarchy of Needs"**

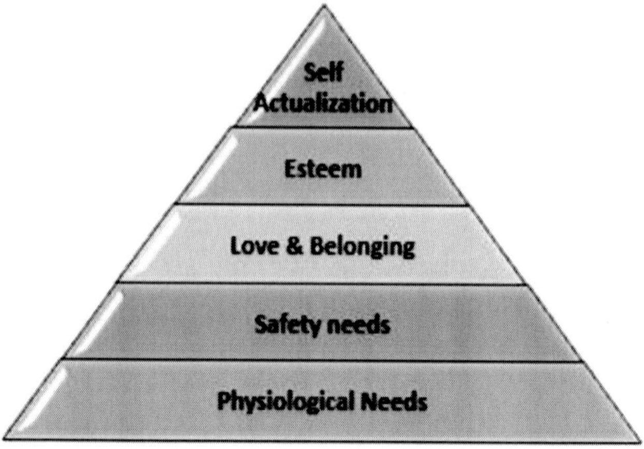

So, whatever problems you are facing is part & parcel in the way to fulfil these needs. The pyramid shape shows that higher needs become important only when lower needs are reasonably met.

The reason why we are running and racing anxiously is actually that We believe happiness lies here, in fulfilment of these needs. But if this is the truth then-

- When you are hungry- and got the food, your physiological need met- you must feel happy till now. Then why again you want to eat your favourite deserts or fast food- And again you get- again you want!
- When you bought a home or got a job- your safety need met- you must be happy till

now- why you are again worried about compliance of your maid, or dreaming for imported furniture, or concerning about EMIs?

- When you got married, and your love and belonging need was fulfilled -you must be happy till now- why you disputed and thought for divorce later?
- When you got first position in fifth standard or got reward in a race competition- your esteem was high- now after not clearing PG why are you feeling failure!
- When you listen to motivational speakers, go in Ashrams to know yourself, spend enough time in spiritual activities and meditation- why again you fall in the pit of sadness and depression?

UNDERSTAND THAT - **THIS IS LIFE PROCESS- IT WILL GO ON THIS WAY ONLY**

WHENEVER A FRAGMENT OF THIS PYRAMID OR ONE NEED IS FULFILLED- IT GIVES YOU PLEASURE- BUT THE NEXT MOMENT THERE IS A NEW DEMAND GENERATED OF ANOTHER FRAGMENT TO

BE FULFILLED- AND IT KEEPS ON GOING- THIS IS THE REASON WHY YOU ALWAYS WANT MORE - THIS ONGOING PROCESS OF DEMAND - DOESN'T LET YOU FEEL FULFILLED

THIS PROCESS IS NOT IN VAIN- IT IS ALSO VERY ESSENTIAL TO MOTIVATE YOU TO KEEP GOING IN LIFE

BUT WHEN YOU SEARCH FOR "ULTIMATE HAPPINESS" HERE- YOU ONLY GETS DISAPPOINTMENT- AS ITS ONLY CAPABLE TO GIVE YOU "MOMENTARY PLEASURES"

So, where happiness is? – where to find it?

my dear- **YOU ARE THE HAPPINESS**

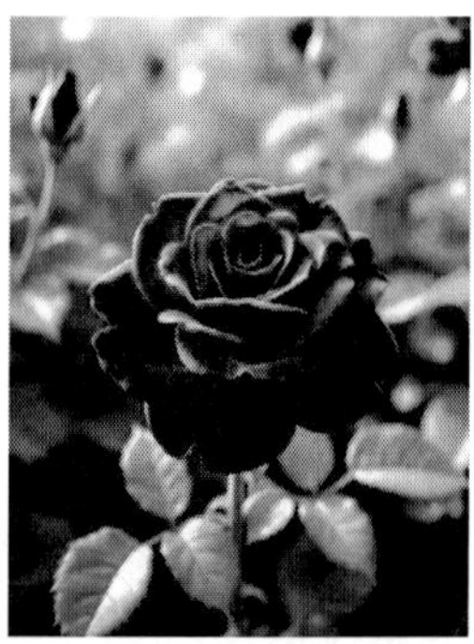

See a Rose- It also have needs in form of water, soil, sunlight etc. which have to be fulfilled in order to continue its life process for which it is also dependent on others.

But they just blossom with full grace, radiating beautiful sight and soft fragrance, making it so pleasant to the soul. In happiness when it blooms, even don't care about thorns; and these "thorns", which are actually prickles, provide a physical defence mechanism to protect them and also support for their growth and help them reach sunlight.

So, here’s the answer with the changed mindset-

A shift from

“Life is not a bed of roses”

to

“Life is a bed of roses, but roses do have thorns”;

And these thorns are actually for our own protection and only help us to grow, as we don’t forget to enjoy the pleasantness of rose because of thorns - likewise don’t forget to enjoy life because of the small hurdles.

Have a belief that every human being, including yourself, is a creation of God, like a flower in the garden, and is good at something. It’s just that someone’s petals are all open, and someone is still a bud who will blossom in their due time in their own way.

You don’t have to win any race, don’t have to be superior to anyone, don’t have to be appreciated by anyone in order to FEEL HAPPY

YOU AS A DYNAMIC LIFE IS THE VERY SOURCE OF HAPPINESS ITSELF

Win race, try to improve yourself, help others, indulge into something creative- but do all this to break the monotony of life- to provide yourself a motivational force to grow- to experience different aspects of life – but not in search of happiness.

Happiness is just here in this moment within you and it always remain there -it's just that you have not explored this truth of life.

Just bloom to your full potential, enjoy yourself, and you are surely going to have-

AN AWESOME EXPERIENCE OF THE WONDERFUL PHENOMENON CALLED AS LIFE

Take a pledge-

HURDLES IN WAY OF FUFILLING NEEDS- CAN'T STOP ME FROM BLOOMING AS A LIFE.

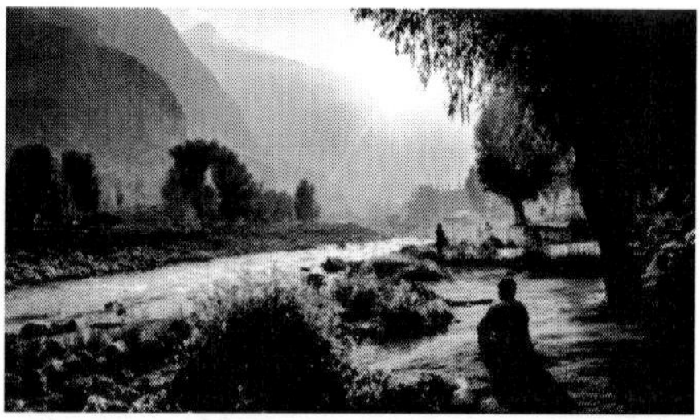

Just look outside; if it's a day… look towards the SUN… yes, it's radiating only for you!!

Even at night, the universe had made arrangements to send some of its light to you…through the MOON….

These stars are twinkling like a hope in the darkest nights.

All the trees, without any partiality, without any biasness, without any favours, are distributing the oxygen which is reaching till you. The beautiful sights of Nature and fragrance of flowers are available for you.

Just evolve your understanding and thought process, know the truths of life, and travel your life's journey with enormous joy, enjoying all these NATURAL BLESSINGS available totally free FOR YOU.

Feel a deep sense of fulfilment — of being alive, aware, and at peace with your journey.

Just blossom & Celebrate growth.

Message from Author

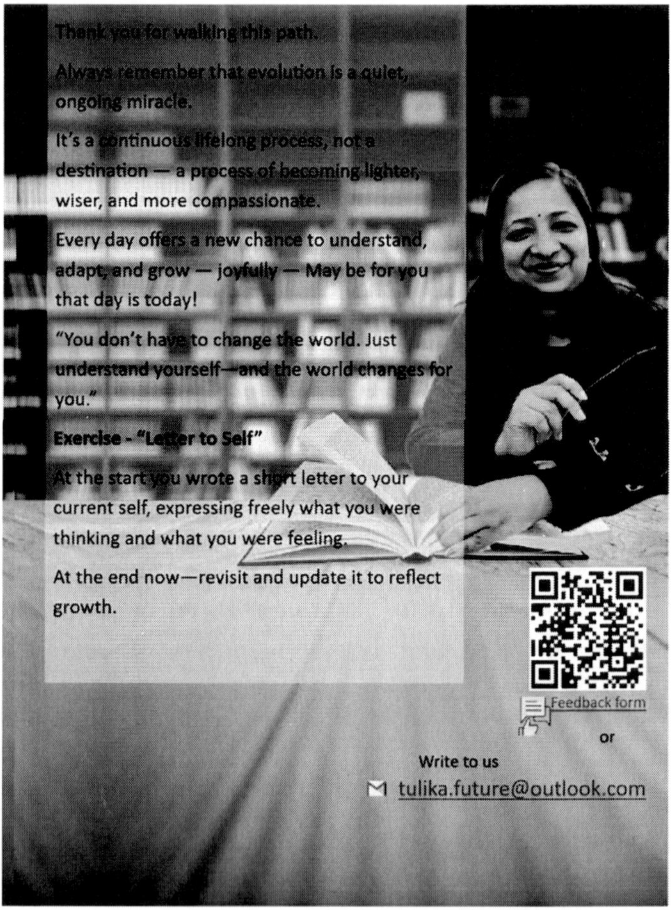